ALLAN JORDAN

GROWING STRONG

The Ultimate Guide on How to Have a Stronger Body, Learn All the Fitness Training and Tactics on How to Become Stronger

Descrierea CIP a Bibliotecii Naţionale a României
ALLAN JORDAN
   GROWING STRONG. The Ultimate Guide on How to Have
a Stronger Body, Learn All the Fitness Training and Tactics on
How to Become Stronger / Allan Jordan – Bucharest: Editura
My Ebook, 2021
   ISBN

ALLAN JORDAN

GROWING STRONG

**The Ultimate Guide on How to Have a Stronger
Body, Learn All the Fitness Training and Tactics
on How to Become Stronger**

My Ebook Publishing House
Bucharest, 2021

CONTENTS

INTRODUCTION

Most medical experts will attest to the fact that some cardio training is better than not having any at all. In order to life a fit and healthy lifestyle one of the prerequisites should be to incorporate some cardio training on a regular basis. Get all the info you need here.

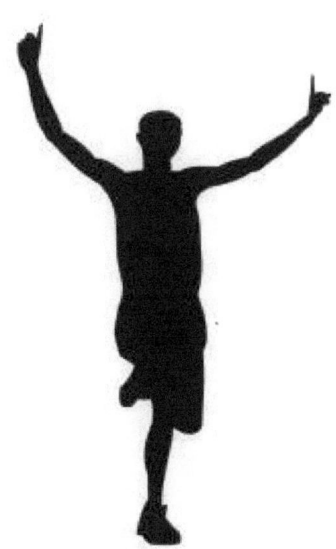

Chapter 1

All You Need To Know About Cardio

It should be noted that there are various types and stages of cardio workouts available for any interested individual. Therefore, some research should be done before the most appropriate regimen it designed and followed effectively. The following are some of the points that should be considered when trying to understand cardio training:

The Basics

Moderate intensity cardio training – for those who are attempting cardio workouts for the specific purpose of getting back into shape or for those who want to put the brakes on the state of obesity currently felt, the moderately designed cardio workout would be more advisable option to start with.

This is mainly due to the fact that most cardio exercises are rather challenging, thus needing the commitment on the part of the participant and if the cardio program chosen is at a difficult level, then the chances of the individual sticking to the program is rather slim. A moderate intensity cardio workout that is done for a longer period of time will give the eventual desired results and will help to keep the individual focused and motivated.

As the desired results become more evident, there may be a need to step up the cardio exercise program to be able to achieve even more form the workout sessions. Putting in more time or more sessions will help the individual gain more muscle mass and lessen the body fat content. Besides this, a more frequent routine would be something healthy to indulge in as opposed to wasting the same amount of time on something that will not benefit the individual.

Chapter 2

Choosing Your Fitness Gear

Choosing the right gear can be a very daunting and confusing task, especially when the equipment available is vast and varied.

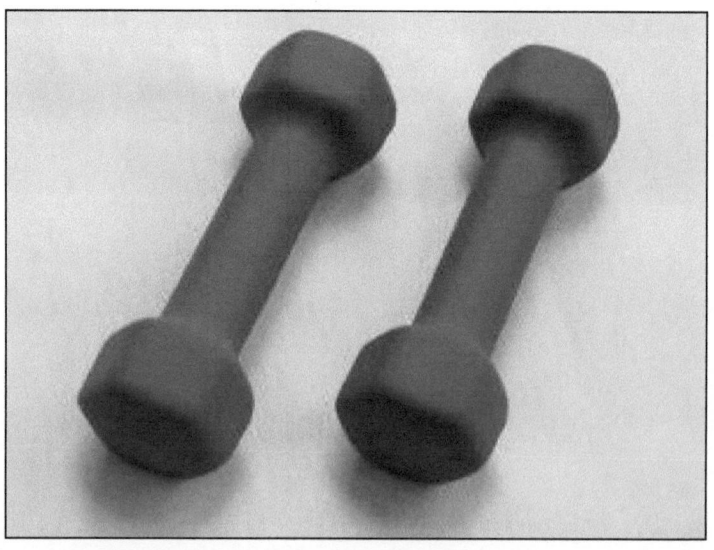

What You Need

For some consulting an exercise expert would be good enough and for others the advice of the sales personnel selling the equipment is something that they would consider.

However, before even embarking on the quest to acquire the suitable fitness gear, the individual should take the time and trouble to define the needs and intentions of the entire exercising foray before the suitable set of equipment can be identified.

There are generally two types of categories the exercises can be grouped into, which the aerobic type and the weight bearing type. The aerobic type, which is also known as cardiovascular training, is meant to raise the heart rate, boost metabolism and put the body into the fat burning mode during the workout sessions.

The weight bearing exercises which is also known as strength training is meant to develop the large muscle groups of the body and increase the muscle mass.

The equipment for the aerobic exercise type would include the treadmills, elliptical trainers, exercise bikes, recumbent bikes, pedal exercises, rowing machines, cross trainers and the stair stepper.

As for the weight nearing type the equipment would most likely include the home gym, work out bench, incline bench, barbells, hand weights or dumbbells, weight sets, weight benches and abdominal exercises.

Although money may also play a large part in the decision for the most ideal fitness gear, the individual should also take into account the long-term usability of the item intended for purchase.

Making a purchase just on the current needs may not be the best choice to make as when the individual has reached the desired phase in the exercise regimen, there may be a need to upgrade the current equipment and this could end up being a rather costly affair.

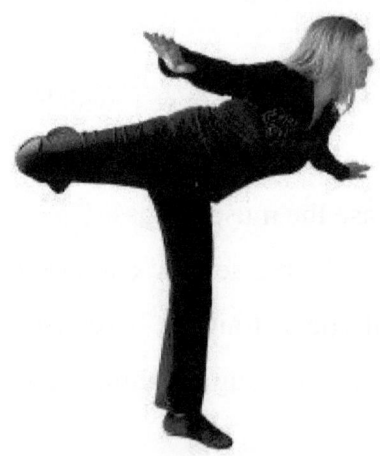

Chapter 3

Your Brain Needs To Exercise Too

Strange though it may seem, there is some real connections between exercising physically and exercising the brain. It is a well accepted fact that the brain becomes sharper and more alert when the individual has a regular exercise routine incorporated into the daily lifestyle schedule.

This is due to the fact that all the positive elements are released in the body systems which then help the brain to function more effectively thus providing the platform for the idea that the brain can and needs exercise to be at its optimum.

Have A Look

Exercising has a positive impact on the nervous system and almost always sets off pleasure chemicals such as serotonin and dopamine which is the ideal ingredient for calmness, happiness and euphoria.

Therefore with regular exercise regimens in place the brain is able to experience all the pleasurable and positive auras, which in turn will allow the brain to think more clearly, perform better and generally sustain a better morale level, thus by stimulating the nervous system the human mind is able to function at a higher level.

When it comes to beating depression, exercise is almost always recommended as here too the chemical released within the body system positively contributes to a better mindset and thought pattern.

A lot of studies have been able to prove the connection between exercising the body and exercising the brain is one and the same. Feelings of anger, fatigue and tension can be dispelled with the appropriate amount of exercise routines if they are done regularly enough.

In fact, some individuals specifically start on an exercise routine anytime they feel any negativity taking over the mind and thoughts. This form of relief has proven its worth for a lot of people.

Therefore, in order to enjoy the feel good mindset and thought process, every individual is encouraged to have some cardio workouts in place on a regular and consistent basis.

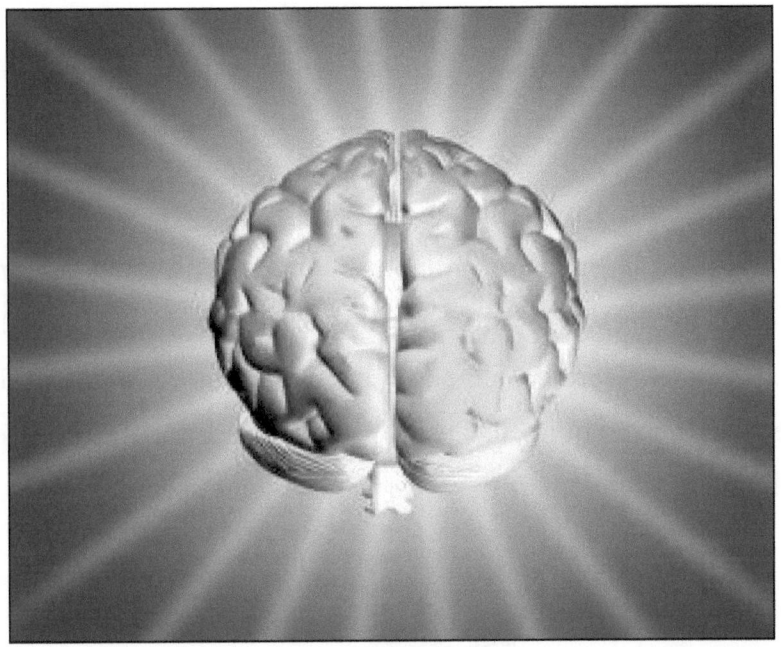

Chapter 4

Cardio Training Regime

There are a lot of different types of exercises that can be incorporated in the cardio training regimen. Understanding and picking the ones that would be most suited to the individual's needs is how a cardio training regimen in designed. Some of the exercises may require the use of certain specifically designed equipment, while others may just require some space.

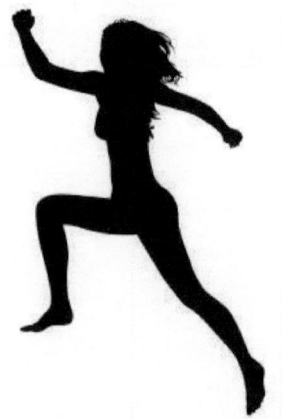

The Workout

The following are some of the more popular cardio training exercises available:

For beginners – this should ideally be done with some very simple and basic exercises done slowly to get the body accustomed to the introduction of the exercise regimen.

The ideal time frame for such workouts should about 3 days of cardio and 2 days of strength training. The cardio training regimen at this stage should ideally include the stationary bike exercise, walking workout, elliptical workout which is all meant to be done within one session.

Alternating this with total body strength workouts or yoga and gentle stretching exercises on other days with the same time frame would generally give the individual an almost complete workout for this stage.

For intermediate – here the similar exercise style is adopted but with a more intense and specific focus on particular parts of the body, and for longer periods of time for each workout session.

Different combinations can be incorporated into the workout but the intensity should be elevated to suit this level and requirements. The workouts should ideally include a 30 minute cardio medley workout, upper body training, and alternating this with 45 minute treadmill workouts and core training. Other days of training regimens may include exercises for lower body workouts and circuit training.

For advanced – here there is more intense focus on immediate training for each individual muscle group to create muscle mass and a toned body.

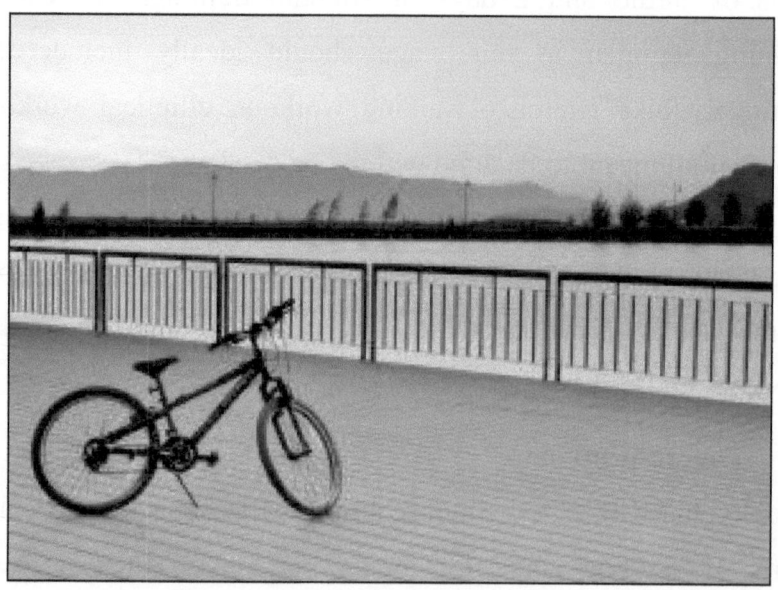

Chapter 5

Stretching Your Body

When it comes to conditioning the body for accommodating exercise regimen, there is a need for the body to be supple, thus the use of stretching exercises. The stretching exercises will help to build the flexibility in the chest, shoulders, back, arms and legs. With the use of a simple set of instruments such as a chair, a ball or a bench, these exercises can commence.

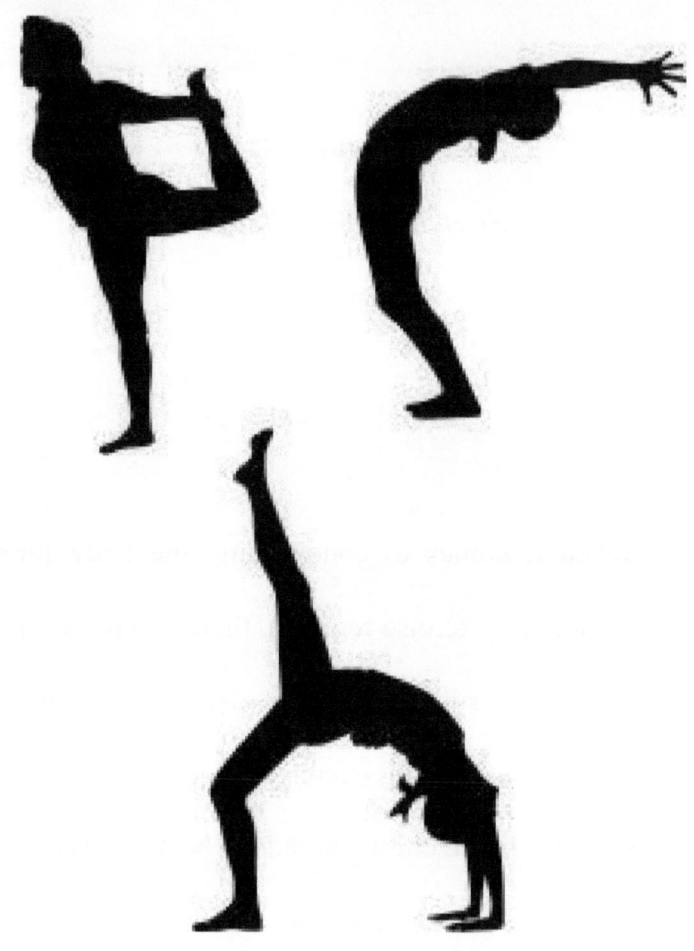

Getting Ready

The following are some example of simple stretching exercises the body can use for conditioning purposes:

Quad stretch – for balance the individual can use a wall and holding on to the right foot the legs should be bent at the knee. Bringing the foot towards the buttocks until the kneecap is pointing straight at the floor.

Hamstring stretch – here the left foot is placed forward and the body is tipped at the hips, while keeping the back flat. Then lower this position until the stretch is felt in the back of the legs. Alternate with the other foot.

Chest and shoulder stretch – sit or stand with the hands clasped firmly together behind the back, while all the time keeping the arms as straight as possible, lift the arms towards the ceiling. This should be done only to a height that is comfortable and the stretch if felt in the shoulders and chest.

Upper back – claps the hands together in front and bend forward enough to create a round back position. Then press the arms outwards until the stretch is felt in the upper back area.

Biceps stretch – stretching the arms outwards with thumbs positioned upwards, and while rotating the thumbs down and back feel the stretch in the biceps.

Shoulder stretch – taking the right arm and placing it straight across the chest, curl the left hand around the elbow area and pull on the right arm gently until the stretch in felt in the upper right arm. Alternate with the other arm.

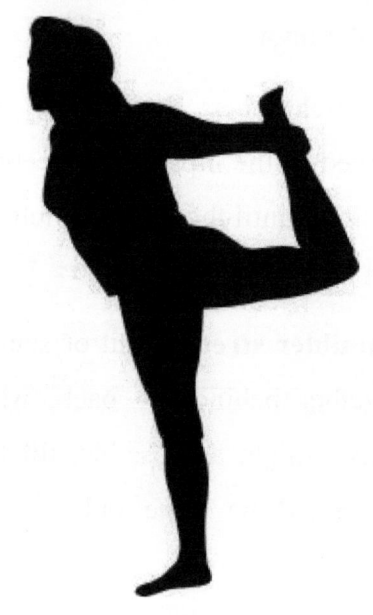

Chapter 6

Handling Injuries

Exercise if done properly is supposed to enhance the general well being of the human body condition. However, it is possible to sustain a number of various different injuries during these exercise workout sessions.

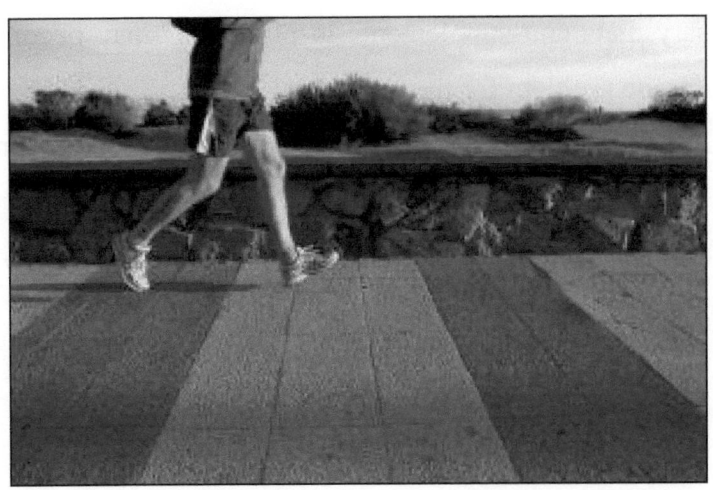

Great Info

The following are some of the tips to help the individual indulging in an exercise avoid possible injuries:

By knowing and recognizing the limitations and the fitness level the individual is capable of, the possibility of sustaining injuries can be avoided as the individual will be able to gauge beforehand if her or she can take on the particular exercise regimen.

Ensuring that the body condition is properly and constantly hydrated is another important element to ensure when working out. The body needs to have the essential vitamins and mineral to function optimally during and after a workout and without the necessary diets and supplements in place, this may become an injury prone problem for the individual.

A lot of people underestimate the importance of proper attire and suitable equipment. With the proper equipment used there is less likeliness of an injury occurring due to the equipment during the workout sessions. Proper attire can also help to prevent blisters and chafing or even causing the individual to be entangled in the equipment.

Adhering to proper warm up and cool down exercises will also help the limit the possibilities of incurring injuries during and after the workout sessions. The mind is more alert and focused thus creating a careful mindset that helps the individual readjust to normal motor movements.

Often people who attempt certain exercises are not really familiar with the actual movements required, and this could lead to injuries being sustained. Therefore, it is very important to get expert advice before attempting any new exercises or unfamiliar equipment.

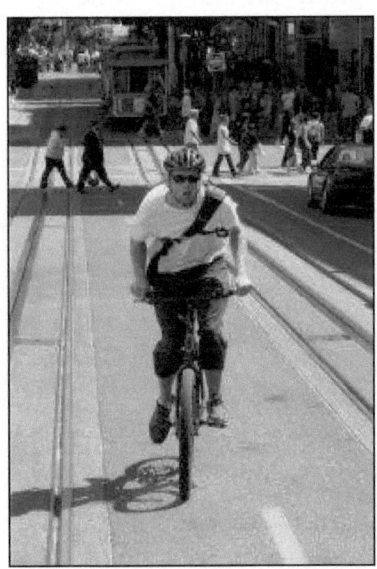

Chapter 7

Watch Your Weight Management

Weight watching is something almost every individual does at one time or another. However, weight watching for those on an exercise program should be done at varied intervals to gauge the effectiveness of the program being followed.

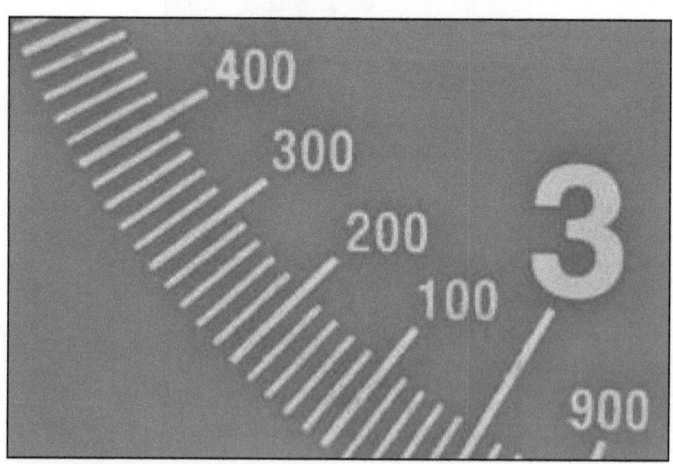

Weight

Sometime the chosen exercise regimen would need to be revamped if the individual is not getting any positive benefits especially in terms of weight loss changes, which should ideally be evident within the first few months of embarking on the chosen exercise program.

There are also other times when it would be necessary to watch the weight progress, and this is especially so if there is a set ideal goal weight that is the focus of the exercise regimen in the first place.

Some people find that watching the weight progress or lack of as a motivating factor. This very visible tell tale sign of the success levels being reached can help to keep the individual focused and willing to continue with the exercise regimen designed.

The weight watching can also help the individual to continue to push for further improvements, once it becomes evident that the exercise regimens are effective.

Weight watching management can also help the individual and those connected to the designing of the exercise program to incorporate exercises that are suitable to the weight of the individual, as this will help to lessen the percentages of possible injury during and after exercises.

The weights would in some cases dictate the kinds of equipment that would be suitable for use without causing undue stress to the body, and this is especially important for those who are just embarking on the exercise routine. Health and weight issues need to be carefully considered for this category of individuals. Thus, the importance of weight watching management should not be underestimated.

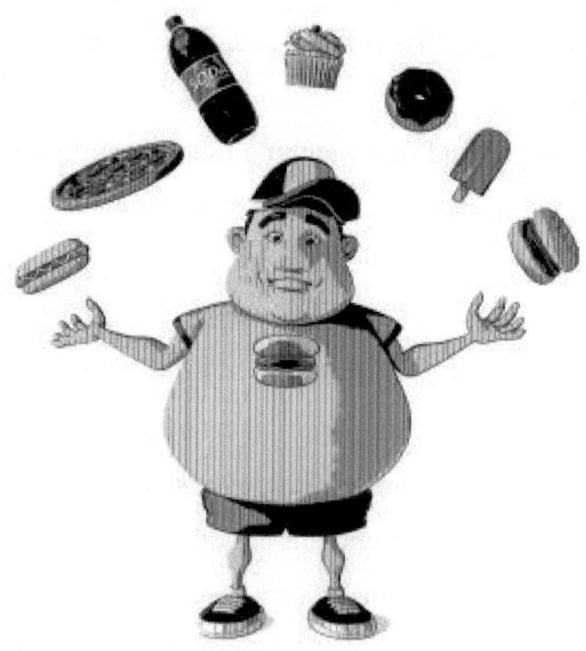

Chapter 8

Watch Your Nutrition

Going on a diet is usually the first step most people take when they want to lose weight of get in shape. This is then accompanied with an exercise regimen that is thought to be suitable for the intended goal.

However, it is very important to understand that when the body feels it is getting a lesser amount of foods it will turn to proteins stored in the muscles to substitute for the lack, instead of breaking down the unwanted fats.

This is the body's way of ensuring the appropriate amounts of energy are still available for the daily functioning of the individual.

What You Eat

Exercise sessions normally demand replenishment in terms of food intake after each intense workout; therefore it would be wise to seek out foods that are both healthy and nutrition such as fresh fruits and smoothies or shakes that are based on healthy content rather than to turn to high fat content foods.

Having a meal before exercising is really not necessary, as it would be very unlikely for a healthy individual to succumb to fainting spells or dizziness due to the regular exercise routine. Having a light nutritious snack would suffice or simply a glass of water. However, for those who have low blood pressure, eating a light meal before a workout session would be advisable.

As the muscles are usually still "feeding" even after the workout sessions have stopped, the ideal time frame to consume a meal would be at least an hour after the exercise. This is to ensure the body does not immediately use the energy provided by the foods consumed leaving the individual hungry again an hour later.

Chapter 9

A Ten Minute Full Body Workout
That Anyone Can Use

When it comes to building muscle, losing fat and getting into shape, the biggest problem for most people is simply sticking to their training goals. This is called 'adherence' in the industry and simply means your ability to stick at a training program long enough to see the results that you need.

Even a poorly designed workout can help you to build muscle and get results if you stick at it. And it is much better to perform a bad workout for a long period of time than it is to perform the best workout possible for a day and then give up.

But this is something a lot of people don't really consider when they plan to get into shape. Too often they will come up with routines that involve training for an hour each session, five times a week. If you're already feeling too tired to be particularly active, if you're already stressed with work… trying to fit in five hours of exercise a week is a huge ask. This is particularly true when you consider that you're probably going to have to travel to the gym as well, get washed, change clothes… etc.

This is where a bodyweight workout can come in so handy. And this is especially true if you use a workout that hits the entire body in a single session, only takes 10 minutes and can be done anywhere. Use this workout first thing in the morning before work and before you go in the shower. Train in your boxers so as to not create more washing.

Now you have a routine that really is just ten minutes and that no one should have any problem sticking with.

What does that workout look like? Here it is:

Three Exercises to Rule Them All

This workout is made up of three exercises that together will train the entire body while also providing some cardio benefit. Those three exercises are:

❑ Pull Ups
❑ Press Ups
❑ Jumping Squats

Perform each exercise to failure and then move straight onto the next exercise when you finish without break. You can rest after the jumping squats for one minute before starting the routine again and going for 3 sets. It should take around 10-15 minutes.

This routine hits all the major muscles in the body because it mimics a more involved split that bodybuilders use called PPL (Push, Pull, Leg). Pull ups hit the lats, the biceps and the abs. Push ups train the pecs, the triceps and the shoulders. And jumping squats hit the entire lower body and provide the cardio.

Now this workout isn't going to be enough to help you build massive muscles overnight. It can burn fat and it can tone your muscles and harden them. But in order for you to really train you need to use heavier weights performed more slowly and for longer.

So use this as a tool to start your new training regime and to get into the habit. Likewise, use it whenever you can't fit a full routine in.

Chapter 10

Gymnastic Rings Are a Fantastic Purchase for Home Gym Owners

If you work out from home, then one of the most incredibly powerful pieces of kit you can buy is gymnastic rings.

Gymnastic rings are rings attached to straps that can hang from your pull up bar. From there, they then enable you to perform dips, inverted push -ps, bodyweight rows and much more. They do everything that TRX does in other words – and more seeing as TRX isn't good for dips – but they cost a fraction of the amount. You can get them on Amazon for $20-40! Plus, they're easy to pack away when not in use and can be taken with you on holiday or anywhere else.

Take a look at some of the things you can do with gymnastic rings for inspiration and to demonstrate just how powerful and versatile they are.

Dips

One of the most obvious things you can do with rings is the dip. A dip simply involves gripping one ring in either hand and then gradually lowering yourself in the middle. This is an excellent way to train the pecs, shoulders and triceps and it also requires a lot of balance and stability.

What's interesting about dips is that you actually can't do them as well on TRX – despite it costing a lot more!

Flyes

You might not have expected this but you can actually perform flyes using gymnastic rings. All you need to do is to lean forward holding one in each hand with your arms apart in a cross position. Now bring them together in the middle to push your bodyweight back up. This is an excellent way to train your pecs and your grip at the same time.

Pull Ups

Using rings to perform pull ups is quite a lot different from not using rings. That's because this has your hands facing inward which makes it a neutral grip pull up instead of a regular pull up. As a result, you'll hit the lats at a different angle, while the wobbly nature of the rings will force you to engage your stabilizer muscles to keep the rings steady and prevent your body from rolling.

Inverted Push Ups

Inverted pushups are surprisingly not a form of push up... but rather another form of pull up! The reason they have this name is that they are effectively push-ups turned upside down. Here, you'll hold onto the rings which are dangling a bit lower and then perform pull ups for your upper body only, with your heels resting on the floor. This allows you to lift a smaller amount of weight during pull ups, which thereby trains your lats but also allows you to use this as part of a drop set. In other words, perform as many regular pull ups as you can, then switch to this to carry on.

Lunge

Performing a lunge with one leg looped into a gymnastic ring is a great way to make it a lot more difficult. This requires more balance again and stimulates the production of more growth hormones as a result.

Chapter 11

Other Forms of Exercise
That Incorporate Bodyweight Training

Bodyweight training has a great number of advantages. This is a way to work out that will allow you to increase your 'strength to weight ratio' thereby becoming more agile, more acrobatic and more powerful. You'll be fast like a coiled spring and strong in a functional way that equates to real-world usefulness.

But there's no such thing as a perfect training modality. And one of the biggest complaints you'll often hear from people who use bodyweight training is that they don't like it because it's 'boring'.

Doing press ups can get old fast and unfortunately just isn't quite so challenging or exciting as lifting 100K over your head.

It doesn't turn heads in quite the same way and the progress can often feel a lot less rewarding.

But that's why it's such a good thing that you can use bodyweight training as part of a more fun or interesting activity or even sport. Let's take a look at some of the great ways you can incorporate bodyweight training into your routine without it feeling like a dull workout. Here are some great examples...

Rock Climbing (Bouldering)

Rock climbing is one of the most fantastic bodyweight workouts there is and it's incredibly fun and rewarding whether you're going to do it seriously or just as a fun hobby. Rock climbing involves using your forearms and grip strength in order to cling to the tiny cracks in the rocks and this can quickly build you Popeye-like proportions.

From there, you'll then be using your lats and your biceps to pull yourself up the wall and scale it like Spider-Man. Better yet, you'll also be holding yourself in position for long periods of time using your legs alone. This quickly builds a lot more quadriceps and hamstring strength so that you'll be getting a truly full body workout.

Bouldering is a great way to get started with this. Bouldering effectively means that you're climbing smaller rocks that present a challenge for how to get to the top. There's no rope and you use a crash mat – so you can turn up at a climbing center and just get started!

Other Forms of Climbing

Don't have a climbing center near you? Not sure you fancy the idea of climbing up the nearby cliffs? A great alternative is something called 'traversing' which is essentially sideways rock climbing. Here you never get that high up and as a result you don't need a rope. As long as you have some kind of natural cliff or wall you can try it yourself!

Or how about climbing a tree? Hand Balancing

Hand balancing is a lost art that is highly rewarding and challenging. Being able to go from a pike position to a handstand requires a ton of muscle power and control, as well as balance. When you pull it off though, you'll have a party trick that's far more impressive than lifting 100 KG and that you can actually do at a party!

Why Bodyweight Training Outdoors is the Ultimate Workout

A word that gets thrown around a lot at the moment when it comes to working out is 'functional'. What is 'functional'? Well essentially, this term refers to the idea that some types of exercises provide real-world and usable strength, whereas others do not.

One of the exercises often called functional is the deadlift because it involves squatting down to pick something heavy up off of the ground using all the muscles in the leg in unison as well as muscles in the back. We pick things up off the floor all the time in real life and every moment is compound in this sense – meaning that we use all the muscles together rather than in an isolated fashion.

An exercise that isn't functional is the bicep curl. Or at least that's how the story goes.

Except that's not quite true in reality. Because in the wild, how often would you actually be required to pick up a perfectly cylindrical bar with perfect technique from standing? Never.

The only times we'd have lifted things in the wild it would have been the carcass of our prey or a boulder we intended to use. The rest of the time our muscles were used for running and climbing and fighting.

And guess what? We never used correct technique. We'd have grabbed things off the ground at an angle and landed awkwardly. And we'd always have gotten back up.

What's more is that we'd never have done the precise same movement more than once. Every time we picked up something, we'd have been at a different angle and the item would have been differently shaped.

And this is why training outdoors with bodyweight is the perfect solution.

How to Keep Challenging Your Body

As soon as you move a press up from indoors to outdoors it becomes more difficult. Suddenly you're training on uneven terrain and one hand will be slightly higher than the other. At the same time, you'll be training in the cold and your lungs will be working harder to supply oxygen.

The same goes double for doing a pull up from a tree branch. Every branch is a different width, meaning you have to use different amounts of grip strength and one hand will always be higher than the other.

You can make this tougher too by lifting logs and doing other non-bodyweight exercises.

But to start with, your usual bodyweight routine moved outdoors is more than enough. And this alone will be enough to start building up a lot more toughness and resilience in your muscles, as well as much more useable strength and power.

And once you start doing this enough, you'll find that you quickly become much hardier and everyday tasks stat to feel a lot easier and less challenging.

Sure, it won't feel very nice at first and you'll get muddy and cold. But that's the point! It's time to stop being domesticated and to get a little wild!

Chapter 12

The Complete Guide to Building Awesome Abs

Abs are the one muscle group that almost everyone wishes they had and that almost everyone wants to make more impressive. The abs are often considered among the 'sexiest' muscle groups and are a sign that a person is slim, toned and athletic. At the same time, building great abs gives you strength and performance benefits that can bleed into every other aspect of your physical ability. That's because the abs provide your core and give you the strength to stabilize yourself during other movements.

But the problem is that many people have no idea how to go about building their abs. With that in mind then, read on and we'll explore what makes the difference between a six pack and a beer belly.

Body Fat

The first thing to recognize is that you need to reduce your body fat percentage if you're going to have visible abs. You can have the strongest muscles possible here but if you don't lower your body fat percentage, then they still won't be visible.

Note that you can't target fat loss. This means that one of the most important keys to building visible muscle here is to make sure that you incorporate CV in order to burn fat as well.

Engaging the Abs

Another thing to recognize is that you need to actually engage your abs during exercise. Many people will perform ab exercises but won't actually be training their abs so much as their hips. The hip flexors can perform a very similar job to the abs by folding the body in half but of course they don't have quite the same visual appeal (if you ask most people).

In short, if you are performing sit ups and leg raises so that your body folds at the waist, then it's not training the abs. Instead, you need to actually roll the abs and curl your stomach round through the movements.

The Different Ab Muscles

Making life more confusing is the fact that you actually have multiple different muscles in the mid-section. The 'abs' as many of us think about them (the six pack) are defined by your rectus abdominis – the muscle plate that sits on the front of your stomach and has the six indentations we all want to achieve.

Meanwhile though, you also have the transverse abdominis. The purpose of this muscle is to provide support for the lower spine and also to 'hold in' the stomach. Training this muscle is not only important for performance, it also helps you to create flatter abs. You can hit this muscle by using the myotatic crunch (a crunch performed over a bosu ball so that your back goes past flat) or by using the 'cat vomit' exercise that involves sucking your abs in while on all fours to create an 'ab vacuum'.

Finally, you have the obliques. These sit on either side of the rectus abdominis and give you more definition here as well as the ability to torque. Train them using twisting sit ups and similar movements.

Training the legs is something of a hot topic among bodybuilders and athletes. Gym goers who 'skip leg day' are often referred to unfavourably and for good reason; training the legs has knock-on benefits throughout the entire body whereas leaving them out tends to make you look disproportioned and odd.

The question then is why so many people leave legs out of their routine in the first place. And the answer is a) legs are boring and b) legs are hard to train.

The simple fact of the matter is that your legs don't have hands attached to them. And this means it's harder to pick up a weight, thus meaning you have to load yourself up some other way and involve the whole body. That instantly reduces the number of exercises available to you and means that leg exercises necessarily take up more space and leave you a lot tireder.

And it also makes it much harder to train your legs with bodyweight alone. But there are ways. Read on to discover some of the best of them…

Jumping Squats

One of the simplest ways to train your legs with your bodyweight alone is to use jumping squats. This simply means that you're squatting down and then jumping at the apex. This is a simple exercise and you wouldn't think that it would make a huge difference – but it is great for building up power and can quickly create a burn thanks to the amount of acceleration involved.

Box Jumps

Speaking of which, box jumps require even more power to launch you high enough into the air – especially if you stack them high. This is in some ways just as challenging as a squat and a great way to build hamstrings, quads, calves and hips.

Jumping Lunges

This is simply a lunge where you jump, switch legs in mid-air and then land with your legs in the opposite position. Doing this is a great way to build strength in the hamstrings and again involves jumping to create more acceleration.

Lunge Walking

Simply walking by stepping from one lunge into the next. This is a surprisingly effective workout because you're plunging so deep in between and spending the majority of your time under tension.

Single Leg Squat

Another way to make the squat more challenging with just body weight is of course to do it on just one leg. This then requires twice the strength and also forces you to balance a lot as well. A more advanced version is the 'pistol squat' which requires your foot to be flat on the ground while the other one is pointed straight out in front of you, toes facing up.

Side Squat

This is between a squat and a lunge and involves stepping out to one side, lunging deep and then stepping back to the middle before repeating on the other side.

Sissy Squat

Finally, a sissy squat is a squat you perform by leaning back and going up on your toes. Your knees point forward and you lean back like Neo. This is tough on the joints so more of a party trick to be used sparingly!

Wrapping Up

It may be rather surprising to note that exercising without the proper nutritional intake is not going to produce the desired results. Most people are unaware that exercising alone without the proper nutritional intake both before and after the exercise sessions will actually be counterproductive. Therefore, it is important to identify and use the proper nutrition when embarking on an exercising regimen.

Printed by Libri Plureos GmbH in Hamburg,
Germany